I0844839

The act of orgasm:
Explore your sexual prowess

Judy o Allen

Acknowledgement

I want to thank my husband, Allen Adamson. He was the one who took me through the process of orgasm. I love him more than I can actually Express in words and am every day genuinely amazed I get to spend my life with him. I try to let him know how much I appreciate him, as often as I can. This is me letting the rest of you to know how to also through this book experience an amazing orgasm because someone taught me how to enjoy sex and not endure it.

Introduction:
orgasming is amazing

I was 15 when I had my first sexual encounter. Prior to then, I had foreplay with my partner, which included kissing, general body contact, and breast stroking. This continued for almost a year. Stupid me! I was just starting off! That seemed to me like sex. Was I enjoying it, you ask? Yes, I was. Actually, I had no idea what I was doing.

This continued until one day my boyfriend took the time to tell me how much joy I would have if I let him inside my vigina. Hmmm. I was terrified! I was unable to simply picture the pain I would experience. After much persuation, I decided to give it a trial. I gave him permission on one of our romantic dates, and then BOOM! Though I didn't know what orgasming was, I was dismayed to discover that the long-awaited pleasure had finally arrived. Wao! I questioned whether I had been missing this all along.

Once more, I believed I was enjoying every aspect of sex. I wasn't, though. More than that was present. I just ended my relationship with the man who first introduced me to the sensation of having his penis pierce my vigor.
I eventually found a much better mate. He guided me through the orgasmic techniques and advice.

I went to see him one day, and we got into our customary romantic position. As soon as his penis entered my vigina, I knew something unusual was about to happen.

We fucked like never before, and I eventually felt like I had a power electric running through my body. My heart also began to beat more quickly, and my body began to vibrate. I told him to fuck me harder, suck my breast, I love you, and I wanted to come at that moment because I believed I was going to urinate. BOOM! It was a GORG!
Wao! I just had the most beautiful and amazing sex ever.

You must realize that in order to have orgasm, you must first visualize and desire it; only then will you be able to enjoy all the desired sexual gratifications.
It's not your lack of experience preventing you from having the finest sex; rather, it's likely that you haven't considered having

the wonderful side as opposed to simply the excellent.

Many of us are not even aware of how little pleasure we are now receiving. Our entire existence has been based on sabotaging pleasure and depriving ourselves of it. Before I discovered the process of orgasming, I was actually performing sex incorrectly.

But if you want to make sex enjoyable in a long-term relationship or you want to feel more confident in the bedroom, there are numerous things you can do without going crazy. Just give these tactics a try.

One of the challenges that married and devoted couples have is how to keep the fires glowing, so to speak, in their sexual lives. Sometimes a couple's sexual loses its passion because they become too used to one another. On the other side, some relationships struggle because the passion or the excitement they once had for one another has faded. What ought you to do in such a circumstance?

Basically, you need to learn how to enhance your love life or relationship, which also entails learning how to enhance your ability to make love.

The importance of sexual intimacy in most relationships outweighs all other considerations. If you want to have a lasting relationship. Don't be afraid to try new things and go back to your old ways! You sure boost your sex prowess by using the heartwarming methods and tips in this book.

Grab a cup of coffee and relax while I take you on a tour into the world of orgasmic.

As you buy this book, my mission is to take you through practical strategies of having a heaven on earth orgasming.

Chapter 1
Simple rules to having a fantastic first-time sex

Since most people find their first experience to be awkward and nerve-wracking, it may not be wise for all of us to try to make it memorable.

A study found that those who lose their virginity and enjoy both emotional and physical fulfillment have more happy sexual lives than those who experience anxiety. The study also revealed that strong emotional bonds form in couples who feel loved by their spouses, whereas sexual sadness might strike those who are less pleased. According to the study, having your first sexual experience is crucial for both your emotional and physical wellbeing.

So, we decode some straightforward advice on how to make it unforgettable.

How to have unforgettable sex

Eating good food is important for your sexual wellness. Ensure that before your first-time sex, you eat healthy and avoid binge eating. Also, if you exercise, you will make your pelvic muscles strong and relaxed that will help in lasting sex for a longer duration.

Don't rush: The most important tip for all you first-timers is don't rush and be patient. Explore your partner. Going slower will make you last longer. Also, as you will be indulging in sex for the first time, rushing may hurt you both

Let her take time: You must be aware that women require more time to reach orgasm than men do. Allocate lots of time for foreplay before allowing her to experience the climax. This will preserve your sexual health while also making your first date with your companion unforgettable.

Look for the sign: While you're busy kissing and cuddling your partner, watch for the appropriate cue that will allow you to make the first move. To avoid injuring your spouse, make sure she is completely excited before applying pelvic pressure on her clitoris

Assess the g spot*:* It will guarantee memorable sex to repeatedly stimulate this unique pleasure organ.

Do you want to be the finest possible lover? If so, then keep reading to learn how to run a marathon in bed while making her scream with need

Her g-spot is optimally positioned when her vagina is appropriately tilted, which eventually cuts down on the amount of time spent in foreplay.

Use a wedge if you want to make sure she's always at the appropriate angle. If that is not possible, you can target her g-spot with other positions; however, the wedge only makes it simpler; or place pillows beneath her pelvic area.

Depth: Since the majority of women's vaginal openings are more sensitive in their outer region, you can tease her by inserting and removing your penis from her opening.

If you look closely, you'll note that in adult movies, the man's penis is never fully extended; some would say that this is simply a function of the camera angle, but it's not.

The G-spot is only approximately 2 inches in, so your penis head can tease her more regularly.
Thanks to the adult film stars' use of this tactic to appease the woman they are having sex with.

Since it isn't a full-on enjoyment of your entire shaft, this can also aid in delaying ejaculation.

One of the kinkiest techniques to induce orgasm in her as well as for yourself is to blow bubbles onto her erogenous areas. Take some pop or champagne in your mouth, depending on your preference, and then smack her.
Once you've done that, press your lips against her clitoris, slowly close your mouth while opening it.
Once you've done that, flick your tongue on her clitoris while still being pressed against her skin, and the fluids will bubble up just next to your tongue.

She can also do this to the top of your penis afterward, and you'll find it so sexy that you'll do it every night.

Additionally, you at least have a unique palate to try cunnilingus with! For evoking feelings, anything effervescent like pop or champagne works wonders.

Most people consider body language to be an essential component of communication. You can converse better and identify romantic interest with the aid of it.

Understanding another person's thoughts or sentiments can be difficult to do by simply seeing or "reading" their body language. Everybody uses body language in their own unique manner, and various sexualities and identities are attracted to others in different ways and to different degrees.

No matter how obvious someone's body language may seem to be, until you talk to them about it, you cannot know what they are thinking or feeling. Therefore, it's crucial to discuss romantic relationships in order to have express verbal consent. Don't skip this stage just because you can see signs of psychological interest in someone's body language.

According to some study, gender may have an impact on how well we "read" body language. It could also affect the way we communicate our attraction.
For instance, some research suggest that those who identify as masculine are historically more likely to demonstrate attractiveness through assertive body language and conduct. Female-identifying people, on the other hand, are more inclined to do so by displaying indications of submission.

Nevertheless, regardless of biological sex, gender identity, or sexuality, many people share features of body language attraction. Furthermore, gender is a continuum and some people may have a fluid gender identity, switching between identifying as male and female. Therefore, even if we might observe whether particular body language signals of attraction are more frequently displayed by men or women, these distinctions probably won't hold true for everyone you meet.

Body language to watch out for.

Lip Licking

A person could feel uneasy when they are around someone they find beautiful. The salivary glands may become active or the mouth may get dry when one is anxious. And both of these incidents can make a person lick their lips.

2. Split Lips

Some people are more inclined to separate their lips (as opposed to licking them) when they are attracted to someone. When your faces are close together, it might be an indication of little apprehension or that they're looking forward to a kiss.

3. Movement of Hips

It's possible to tell someone is attracted to you by the way their hips move. For instance, while music is playing, slight hip movements might indicate that someone is at ease and might be interested in you. To express attraction, people may also touch their partner's hips.

4. Face And Eye Movements
A powerful indication of emotions, including desire, may be seen on the face. For instance, if someone is drawn to or linked to you, their facial expression can resemble yours. Or, their face could exhibit expressive features like a smile, arched eyebrows, or sporadic eye widening.

A person who finds you attractive may also make an effort to make eye contact with you, albeit how long it lasts will depend on their personality. They may even scan the whole body of the person they are drawn to, allowing them to see everything

5. Smile.

Another way some individuals display their openness when dating is through smiling. When you smile and show interest in someone, you might appear more approachable and appealing.

Advice for successful flirting in the dating world

1: adoringly and observing. We all struggle to look away when attracted to someone. The lusty stare continues even after the object of our lust has stopped speaking. Use this as an opportunity to be a little provocative and, during a gap in the talk, keep your eyes on your date for a silent count of five. In contrast, your date will blink more frequently if they are feeling anxious.

2: Hands. Anxiety and tension are indicated by clenched fists, hands that are tightly knit, or hands that are placed against the mouth. Even worse is if their hands are supporting their heads, as this either indicates complete ennui or that they are going to pass out from exhaustion or drink. People who are anxious may fidget with things on the table or grip their own hands. Open hands on the table with the palms facing up imply a more laid-back and approachable individual. If you're feeling extremely anxious, consider placing your hands loosely clasped on the table; this projects less anxiety than clutching your fingers or folding your arms. Speaking while placing your hands on your chest gives the impression that you are vivacious and sincere.

3: Speech volume. Their tone won't be too high or too low if they view you as their equal. Strong personalities often have loud voices, while meek types tend to have gentle voices.

4: Unintentional autoerotic touching. We unconsciously touch ourselves as a result of sexy thinking for a variety of reasons. In the beginning, to draw attention to different bodily parts. Girls will rub their upper arms, thighs, hips, and waists, while guys will both stroke their lips. Second, we poke fun at one another by touching ourselves. Thirdly, everything becomes extremely sensitive when one is sexually excited because blood is racing around the engorging extremities. Once touched, it feels good.

5: Mouth. When your date begins to eat, drink, or smoke more quickly, this is a highly strong sexual body language gesture. You reach for your mouth while you are thinking about sex. Putting objects in your mouth could indicate that you have a sexual curiosity. Girls play with spoons, lick ice cream cones, and suck their fingers.

6: Her Hair. Girls that are interested begin to play with their hair. The strongest of all hair flicks, hair fluffing, and caressing are all signs of availability or flirtation in body language. But if she starts to cower behind her hair, that's a sign of disinterest.

7: **Fiddling Guys.** Guys begin to emit their own flirtatious signals as their sexual excitement increases. He might toy with his tie, touch his nose, slide rings over his fingers, or fiddle with some loose change in his pocket. He is trying to look good for you if he is adjusting his hair.

8: Examining your butt. When you leave the table to go to the bar or the bathroom and you catch your date looking at your butt, they are probably thinking lustfully.

9: **Stripping off symbolically.** Strong sexual body language gestures include removing jackets, loosening ties, undoing buttons, and pushing up sleeves. Mother Nature's method of getting us naked with someone we have a sexual chemistry with is to unconsciously undress in public.

10: Touching. Uncertain where the date will go? Test your touch. Touch their shoulder, arm, or hand. If they like you, they should touch you back within ten minutes, barring shyness.
There should be three sets of touching for a total of three seconds on a good first date.

11. Wineglass. If he is wiping the rim of his glass with his fingertips, the date is a success. The same applies if she moves her glass up and down. She is undoubtedly flirting if she is also making eye contact and fiddling with her straw. Wine glasses held at chest height or higher, however, are a hint that a second date won't happen. Similarly, if your date puts both of their hands around their glasses wineglass examination. This is a fantastic test of subliminal body language to evaluate that first date. Start having fun with something on your side of the table, like a wineglass or a spoon. Gently shift it over to your date's side of the table while you lean forward a bit. Lean back, take your hands away, and continue speaking. If your date pushes it back to you carelessly, they are not interested. You're in luck if they hold it or leave it where it is. Push something else in their direction and keep your arms on the table to advance the conversation. The astute date will now lean forward and shove something toward you from their side of the table.

12: A hearty kiss. Touching their mouth, licking their lips, moving their head close to yours, eating and drinking seductively, and tilting their head while looking at you are all clear indications that your date is open to a kiss.

Start the kiss by lightly brushing their lips together. You should stop if they withdraw, clamp their lips, or slap your face. They are willing to go on if you lean forward, part your lips, or touch the back of your neck.

Never before has courting with nonverbal cues been so simple! Use this dating advice to decipher nonverbal cues and project your own sexual cues. the first date into a second date via flirting

Chapter 4

Beyond the female G-spot is the U & A spot.

The G-Spot, which was first identified by Grafenburg, has been the subject of a lot of writing. A portion of a woman's vagina that, when stimulated, may produce tremendous pleasure is this one.

The human body is now disclosing more of its secrets because of advancements in non-invasive anatomical examination using MRIs, CAT scanners, and other extremely sensitive investigative tools.

Here, we'll look into two recently found pleasure zones that are located in the general genital zone of women.

"The U-Spot."
The U-spot is a tiny patch of extremely delicate erectile tissue that is situated above and on either side of the urethral opening.

The stimulation of this aera by the tongue, the penis, or even a greased finger caused an unexpected and extremely potent sensual reaction, according to some American clinical researchers who recently identified it. This is the area just above and to the side of the urinary entrance.

There isn't a U-spot extending from the urethra to the vagina. When attempting to excite it, use caution and get input from your partner.

The Anterior Fornix Erogenous Zone (AFE) is sometimes referred to as the T-Spot or the A-Spot.

The AFE Zone technically speaking, is a hub of nerves that transmit data from your whole genitalia to your spinal cord and brain. These nerves, when activated, convey arousal signals to the area of your neurological system that improves engorgement of the proper locations and is subsequently in charge of causing sexual excitement.

The same is true for females who are often not sexually receptive.
Naturally, the simplest approach to detect the AFE zone is to slip your fingers halfway up the posterior vaginal wall. You will find a

wider region than the G-spot, which is a little rougher than the usual vaginal wall.

The location Of the g spot

The male g spot is situated on the top wall of the anus, facing the front of the body, roughly 1 to 2 inches deep. Unlike the female g spot, it is not a specific place but rather a region that may be stimulated. When you touch the male g spot, you will experience unusual and potent feelings.

Guidelines For A Male G Spot Orgasm

Dry orgasms need complete surrender and relaxation to the energy.

Additionally, moving the energy involves making noises and taking deeper breaths from the abdomen

How to stimulate the male g spot
If you want your spouse to be comfortable, start with a good sensuous massage. When you both feel ready, move on to stroking their prostate externally. It's simpler to lie him on his back and use your index and middle fingers to touch, rub, stroke, or push his perineum (the region of skin from under his testicles to his anus), experimenting with different pressures and feelings. To further arouse him, stroke several different areas of his body with your other hand.
As the massage is just started, ask your spouse what he finds relaxing.

Once your partner is relaxed, insert your finger(s) about an inch or so into the area and glide them upward along the side of the rectal lining that faces his front. Look for a little, spherical tissue bulb; this is the prostate. Once you've found it, make a "come here" motion with your finger(s). Keep in mind that the prostate gland is a highly fragile organ and should always be handled with care.

Take his penis in your hand or mouth while you massage his g spot. Some men may experience orgasms after prostate stimulation alone, but the majority require additional stimulation

Does Size Matter?

On whether having a big, lengthy penis is advantageous or disadvantageous, there has long been disagreement. No matter how big a man's penis is, in the case of the AFE zone, he needs experience to locate and stimulate the AFE zone.

There are certain advantageous postures for the male with a shorter penis to shorten the woman's uterus and yet stimulate the AFE zone.

Even if he is short and little of penile size, the advanced missionary will completely penetrate and stimulate the AFE zone by having the woman's legs brought to her breast, keeping her legs apart with his arms, and hanging himself from her.

Self Penis Enlargement (SPE) Technic
The secret to giving ladies the most unforgettable sexual encounter of their lives

is often a larger penis size. Here are some suggestions for men who are stuck trying to figure out how to increase the size of their penis.

Penis exercise. Penis exercises are the most efficient approach to increase penis size and girth size with little expense and long-lasting effects. Men could improve in bed and increase their self-confidence and self-esteem by getting a longer, thicker penis.

The jelq method and PC flex exercises are perhaps the most efficient. Your initial priority should be to improve the flow of blood through your penis during an erection. Always begin your workout with a warm-up exercise in which you simply wrap your penis around a warm towel for one to three minutes.

Your penis will get longer and thicker if you boost blood flow to the muscles that support it. This will also encourage the development of new cells and tissues.

Like every other muscle in your body, your penis is a muscle. Like your biceps or abdominal muscles, it can be strengthened through exercise. It's not hard to enlarge your penis size and girth even if you were born with a smaller package. Your blood circulation will improve, which is crucial for getting better erections that will make your spouse more satisfied while you're in bed.

 Tip. There are several exercises you can perform in the privacy of your room to enlarge your penis. Only a damp, warm towel and a lubricant like KY Jelly, Vaseline, or any other lotion, oil, or petroleum jelly would be required. Put the warm cloth on your penis for a minute, wipe it off, and then gently pat and stroke it till it becomes semi-erect to erect. When the penis is sufficiently erected, oil it with the lubricant of your choice and grip the shaft with your thumb and pointing finger wrapped around it. This process is known as milking. As though you were milking a cow.

Pull the penis slowly till it is fully extended. Be sure to continue this until you are still feeling at ease or satisfied with the act. Perform the pulling and tugging motion 25 times. This is regarded as penile workout as well. As long as you use the milking technique, you are free to continue masturbating. On the 25th count, you can decide to stop. Everything hinges on you. After completing the exercise, reapply the warm cloth to the penis for about a minute. At least twice a day, perform this.

Warning: If you don't perform the penis exercises consistently, you won't see the desired effects as soon as you'd like. This is as effective as any other exercise regimen; if you commit to it and stick with it, you will notice results quickly.

How to dominate the A and U spot

If you want to offer your partner mind-blowing orgasms during a sexual encounter, you must be able to locate her G-spot and stimulate it. She will experience many climaxes in addition to a strong orgasm as a result of this.

Get her excited so that she is hot and eager for you before you can activate her G-spot. Finger stimulation is often used to hit the g-spot. Penile stimulation, however, finger stimulations can trigger the g-spot in various sexes positions. The modified missionary position, the jack hammer, the doggy style, and the postures with women on top are the main positions that promote g-spot stimulation. The doggie style is arguably the most well-liked of these three. You must be angling your penis downward to bump against the g-spot in the doggy position in order to correctly strike it. Your penis shouldn't necessarily be directed vertically, but it should be slightly vertical as it enters the vagina. You can come down straight without being constrained by the woman's buttocks if you elevate your torso and hips above hers.

Positioning the female's buttock with pillows will enable you to shove up toward the g-spot while in the missionary position. Imagine hitting the core of your partner's pubic hair from underneath to help you envision this. The cushions should be adjusted by your spouse to best target the region. Another great posture to use the penis to target the g-spot is with the woman on top. To make this work, you need to be chest to chest, with the male partner pushing into the g-spot while the female partner pushes into the penis, pretending to be attempting to hit below the pubic hair.

The Jackhammer position is one of the least cozy, yet most effective postures for striking the g-spot. The man should essentially be standing above the female with his penis pointing vertically like a jack hammer, while the female should be resting on the top of her back and neck. However, you must approach at an angle when doing the jackhammer with the goal of activating the g-spot. Come from below and above, pressing towards the pubic hair and aiming for the clitoris.

Stimulate the G spot to squeal in ecstasy

To get her warmed up, begin with some lengthy, sensual foreplay. Keep in mind that if you want her to orgasm, do not neglect the foreplay. Then, massage her genitalia while smearing warm lubricants on your fingers. Slide your fingers within her vaginal wall as you become more and more warm and moist. Once you locate a little, bean-like tissue with a bumpy feel, gently rub the entire area. The G spot, or female orgasm's Holy Grail, is there. Normally, it is only 1.5 to 3 inches away from the vaginal opening.

Pushing herself to climax

Once you've located her G spot, perform a come-hither motion against the hot region with your index and middle fingers. Start by applying rhythmic pressure slowly. Then, try varying the tempo and intensity. When you observe one or more of the following on her: quick breathing, groaning, blushing, and the fluids becoming more and more watery, you know you've hit the proper button. If you are unsure, ask her preferences and whether you are acting appropriately.

Pull out your finger and ask her to wait a little while after she starts to become enthusiastic. It's a tactic to "tease" her and heighten the arousal. You will be astounded at how quickly she hits big "O!" as you excite her once again. Next, enter her body from the back or in a cowgirl stance. Your penis might commonly reach the G spot in these positions. To make sure your member touches the G spot, keep thrusting shallow.

It is necessary to excite her first so that she is hot and eager for you before you can activate her G-spot. For help, refer to the advice below:

Warning: Since you'll be using your fingers a lot during sex, please trim your fingernails. You don't want to injure her in her delicate and private parts, unless you don't want to satisfy her. If you need to keep your fingernails short for any reason, wear a laxative. For the best G spot orgasm, you need increase the size of your penis. When the partner is overweight, the pleasure and experience of sex will be enormously enhanced

It is advised that your meal should contain both protein and fiber. Some examples of these foods are yogurt with fresh fruit or peanut butter on whole wheat toast, soya food products (such as tofu or soybean curd), smoked salmon scramble, high protein oatmeal banana chocolate chip mookies (a muffin and cookie combo), vegetables, high fiber fruits (guava, pineapple, green apple, lime, and lemon), low sugar soya milk, low sugar red bean soup, and low sugar barley soup.

You will be able to stay active for the most part because this protein- and fiber-rich food combination takes longer for your body to digest, allowing you to fully enjoy the sensual moment with your spouse.

 Good diet is a necessity it you want to have a fabulous orgasm

It is often much simpler to improve one's sexual life. You don't need to overindulge in such primarily untested aphrodisiacs by medicine. Simply allowing your body to consume a variety of vitamins and nutrients from your regular diet will give you a vibrant sex life. A well-balanced diet is a prerequisite for having a good sexual life.

I'm going to emphasize the six dietary. considerations that you should put in order to boost both your overall health and your love life.

1. Avoid consuming excessive amounts of foods high in refined carbohydrates, such as bagels with cream cheese, refined cereals, cookies, puddings, pasta, custards, processed grains, doughnuts, cakes, candies, soft drinks, and soda, which can quickly raise your blood sugar level before quickly plummeting, leaving you feeling lethargic and lacking in sex motivation.

(2) Fruits and plain water as opposed to sugary, caffeinated beverages
It is good to drink enough plain water to replace any fluid lost when you first wake up in the morning and/or after your typical workout in order to avoid becoming dehydrated. How much liquid is sufficient for you? The color of your urine is the best indicator. If it's yellow, your body still needs more water, so you should drink a few more

glasses of simple water. You can add low-calorie beverages (such green tea, Chinese tea, and fruit juices) and high-water-content foods (including watermelons, limes, red grapes, lemons, carrots, and tomatoes) to this throughout the day.More than two cups of coffee or tea can overstimulate you and make you feel tense even at the end of the day, but one cup can perk up your morning and aid in your ability to stay focused. Avoid consuming excessive amounts of those sugar-rich beverages (natural fruit juice is acceptable) or soft drinks, which can produce huge swings in your blood sugar levels.

(3) **Avoiding red meat and processed baked items in favor of unsaturated fats**. Rigidly adhering to a very low-fat diet can deprive your body of the fats necessary to produce the sex hormones (testosterone, estrogen), which may decrease your desire for sex. One way to fight this is by consuming foods like olive oil, fatty salmon, almonds, and cod liver oil, which are sources of omega-3-rich unsaturated fats. Premenstrual syndrome and postmenopausal heat flashes in women can be avoided with the use of omega-3 fatty acids.

Avoid eating too much red meat, which is high in processed baked goods and trans fats, and processed baked goods that are high in saturated and trans fats. The amount of blood that reaches your genitalia may be reduced or blocked by them.

(4) Choosing lean proteins like chicken, fish, and eggs over high-calorie junk food Eat less of fast food, fried meals (such ad fried potato chips), which can lead to an unintentional buildup of harmful fats in your body and eventually impair your sex drive. Consider melon seeds, low-fat frozen yoghurt, unsalted roasted pumpkin seeds, unsalted roasted sunflower seeds, unsalted roasted peanuts, and unsalted roasted cashew nuts if you feel the want to chew on something or snack out of boredom.

(5) One glass of wine after a meal as against alcohol.
A glass of wine, especially red wine, can improve blood flow,

which is healthy for the heart. It can also calm you and help you feel more open to closeness and romantic gestures. However, consuming too much alcohol might depress your central nervous system, causing you to feel tired and reduce your sex readiness.

(6) Dark chocolate consumption as against eating a big meal before sex. According to a German research that was published in the journal Appetite, chocolate may instantly improve most womenCAghly 90 minutes. Having a large meal, however, may cause your genitals to receive very little blood flow, which might cause your digestive system to be overworked. Here are six nutritional recommendations for a healthy sexual life. In general, what is healthy for your total well-being is healthy for sex. What is excellent for your heart will help you sustain an erection, especially if you're a man.

Food to avoid if you must have a great sexual pleasure

Our sexual health is significantly influenced by our way of life and behaviors. Sometimes, altering our surroundings and our behaviors might increase sexual performance.

For instance, exercise frequently improves our mood, which is beneficial for the bedroom as well. Nutrition is also crucial, and there are several items you shouldn't have on hand.

Other meals to avoid

1. Liquor

Red wine might help establish the mood before having sex, but over drinking is bad for you. Alcohol inhibits the central nervous system, and erections require the central nervous system. As a result, excessive drinking may contribute to erectile dysfunction.

Additionally, drinking might diminish your sex urge. When you drink frequently and heavily, your testosterone levels will decline. Long-term, this lowers libido and leads to various health issues.

2. Sour foods

To maintain good erections, blood flow and blood pressure are crucial. Given this, it is easy to understand why eating salty food is hazardous for your sexual health.

When you consume this kind of meal, your blood pressure significantly rises. On the other hand, blood supply to smaller organs decreases, which has an impact on erections and orgasms.

These meals should be avoided before sexual activity, especially if you have high blood pressure. Your blood vessels will have effects since they won't produce as much nitric oxide. Simply eating better may help certain erectile dysfunction patients.

3. **Cofee**

If you need to wake up and feel more energized, coffee may be helpful. However, i do not advise drinking coffee shortly before having sex. Coffee may increase your blood cortisol levels, according to studies. This stress hormone may make it challenging to unwind.

In addition to having a sexual urge, having an erection requires at least some mental tranquility. Coffee can exacerbate your anxiety and jitteriness if you already have it, and it will lower the quality of your erections. This result might differ from person to person.

4. Dairy Cheese and dairy products should be avoided before sexual activity.

We are accustomed to eating dairy products and having digestive issues.

Thought to be a typical aspect of digestion, it is not. Even if you are lactose intolerant, the symptoms might still get worse. But even if you're not, eating dairy may cause you to feel bloated.

Burping and stomach pains may be devastating sex drive killers. Therefore, we advise saving dairy until another time if your sexual function is your main priority

5. Beans

Similarly, beans should be avoided before having sex for a very straightforward reason. A certain type of dietary fiber found in beans affects how your bowels function. Although this can be advantageous in some circumstances, it is not particularly pleasant when having sex. Being able to feel your bowel motions won't be at all comfortable.

Beans can help lower cholesterol levels and promote cardiovascular health. Just attempt to eat them at a different time.

6. Onions

Onions should not be eaten before having sex due to their strong aroma. It's not because onions are unhealthy for you.

They only make you have foul breath and smell bad. Therefore, you might wish to avoid having onions in your excellent supper if you want to create a special atmosphere.

7. Carbonated beverages.

Avoid any fizzy beverages before the sex begins if you want to have better sex. Belching is the major issue with carbonated drinks once more, and it often occurs one or two cups in.

Additionally, soft drinks might lower your testosterone and harm your libido. They have high sugar content and are linked to metabolic issues and obesity.

Building stronger bonds in every relationship starts with open communication. In a healthy relationship, communication should not be limited to only particular aspects of the relationship but should also include sexual preferences and wants. Communication is key to any good sexual connection. According to research, talking to your spouse about your sexual needs and desires will improve your sex life and strengthen your relationship. The cornerstone of every relationship is trust, which may be developed between you and your partner by being open about your sexual preferences. You should be able to discuss your medical issues, physical issues, any limitations you may have, as well as your likes and dislikes, in order to have a good sexual or nonsexual relationship

When you and your partner are able to convey your needs and wishes without making the talk difficult and while taking into account how the other feels, is sexual communication. It is a rewarding, pleasurable, and enjoyable aspect of life. The vital component of a relationship is the physical side of love, and talking to your spouse about it only strengthens it. You'll find it simpler to have sex safely and have a fulfilling sex life if you have sexual communication.

Physical Interaction: Verbal communication is simply one aspect of communication. Sometimes all it takes to draw someone to you is a little touch on your shoulder or back, a quick glance in your direction, or even a wink. Physical closeness is the primary means of obtaining wonderful, healthy sexual activity. Couples almost always discover what the other is thinking without asking. In this instance, the adage "actions speak louder than words" is amply shown. So make sure you can read each other's body language.

sexual preference. Giving your partner verbal or physical direction during a sexual encounter is essential to having a fulfilling sexual life. To turn you on, he or she has to know where to touch you and where not to. Sexual fulfillment will not only become difficult but also dangerous if your partner has no idea what you could desire or expect in bed. The sexual experience will be 10 times better if you two communicate verbally, such as by saying "kiss me" or "touch me there." Only when there is love and appropriate sexual communication can this occur.

Communication in Conversation: Vocal communication is the sole way to elicit a sexual yearning. Good oral communication is essential to all relationships. It is important to communicate about sex in a way that avoids awkward or unpleasant situations. Numerous problems in your romantic and sexual life will be resolved. You must pay attention to what your spouse could like doing more or how you might avoid or finally fix problems that generate conflict.

Intimacy: Emotional and sexual closeness both demand open communication. While some expose their internal inhibitions, others are cautious in their sexual expression. Every couple has developed their own distinct and distinctive ways of communicating with one other. To be most compatible with your partner, it's critical to be able to express yourself easily and freely and receive immediate feedback from them. You can contact a sexologist and ask a free inquiry if you want to talk about any specific sexual issue.

Keys to effective sexual communication. Sexual action and intimacy need two people to communicate with one another. Greater sexual comfort and enjoyment can result from being open and honest with one another. Many people find it challenging to appropriately discuss sex with partners. When someone attempts to talk about their wishes but is unclear of how to articulate them, there may be some amount of uneasiness that develops.

The following sentences provide details about sexual communication methods.

1. Be Specific

Although it is sometimes challenging, it is crucial to have a clear and precise conversation with a partner before engaging in sexual activity for a number of reasons. Learning about and comprehending one another's limits, wants, preferences, and desires is a part of the continual communication process. Before having sex, being explicit in your *communication might make sexual talk later on simpler.*

A straightforward approach for obtaining consent is the first step in good sexual communication.

Although straightforward communication about permission is crucial, the process of being explicit about sexual behavior involves much more than just responding "yes" or "no." It involves assisting one another in fully comprehending the needs, wants, and aspirations of the other. One may express, for instance, if foreplay is a crucial aspect of sexual activity or if sex toys are desired, and if so, which ones. If both of you feel comfortable doing so, you may also choose to discuss your sexual desires.

Sexual interaction may not necessarily require vocal communication. Body language,

which may be expressed through the eyes, hands, lips, face expression, and body, is another crucial component of communication. You can use terms like "touch here," "touch there," "harder," "softer," "more," "less," "faster," and "slower" to express your sexual wants. All of these phrases may be used to swiftly and effectively express what you want, but they can also lead to misunderstandings, such as when "faster" is taken to indicate "harder." Here, it is crucial to talk openly in order to ensure that both you and your partner have a satisfying time when having sex. It also lets people know when their sexual behavior has to be modified or corrected.

2. Positive attitudepp

The bedroom is not the only place where the golden rule is applicable. Alternatively said, "the golden rule applies in the sheets as much as on the streets."1 When learning about sexuality between couples, these proverbs emphasize the value of kindness, support, patience, and cooperation. Remembering to be patient and upbeat while communicating sexually is essential. Avoid focusing too much on criticism or displeasure. Many people find discussing sexual activity to be quite unpleasant, yet as was already said, communication is crucial to ensuring that both parties have the knowledge necessary to engage in consenting sexual activity.

This part of the Golden Rule is crucial for making accommodations for people with disabilities. It is essential to continue

In order to have open and honest conversation with your spouse during a time when each individual may feel vulnerable, work on being positive rather than negative while speaking with them. By being useful and effective rather than obsessing over something you might not have loved, talk to them and explain why you did not enjoy something. For example, a woman with a handicap may discover that the pressure was either too strong or too gentle, that a particular position hurt, or that there was no pleasure. Being courteous and non-judgmental while discussing these issues demonstrates that you comprehend the other person's perspective. People must respect limits and take into account the needs and desires of their partners.

3. Pay attention and ask questions.

Pay Attention and Ponder

Being able to listen can be challenging since many of us have a tendency to begin formulating our responses while the other person is still speaking, rather than "listening" to them and what they have to say. You must concentrate on your partner's words and give them your whole attention if you want to hear what they are saying. If your spouse tells you, for instance, "I need you to press harder on my clitoris when you are using your fingers during foreplay," they are telling you, "here is how you can make me happy." In order to fully understand what your spouse is saying, it might be beneficial to ask follow-up questions. "So what I hear you saying is..." one illustration.

Vulgarity brings intimacy

Being able to express your own distinct sexual expression may be quite gratifying because sexuality has such a wide range of manifestations.

There is a technique to become more active if you are a shy, introverted lover who believes there must be more to it: Master the art of dirty language and go over your immobility. You turn yourself on in addition to your spouse.

When you send your boyfriend a flirtatious SMS while he is at work, he won't be able to stop thinking about you. It's mental foreplay, which is really hot for maintaining the fire in your relationship. Does it sound okay? Do you agree?

Note:It's more important how you say it, than what you say. Don't focus too much on the words you use, focus on how you say it and on your intention.

How would you feel hearing these incredible vulgar words at the point of orgasming?

 You don't have to say anything in particular during an orgasm. You can continue saying the same things you did during intercourse after you reach your climax. However, there are a few orgasm-specific phrases you may whisper shortly before and during the cum:

Harder!
Suck my breast
I am going to cum.
I'm chewing.
I'm going to orgasm because of you.
(Unable to achieve orgasm? Learn the cause of your inability to orgasm and the remedy.
I am powerless over myself.
Fuck.
I'm struggling so much. If this is your second, third, or fourth time climaxing, I'm going to squirt (learn how to squirt when masturbating and during sex).
God.,Jesus.

Chapter 7
Orgasmtic state

The majority of individuals only understand clitoral orgasms. The reality is that there are several varieties of FEMALE ORGASM. When you start to blow her mind in the bedroom and offer her genuinely GREAT SEX, you'll start to give your partner more than simply clitoral orgasms.

Female Orgasms: Here Are 7 Spectacular Orgasms You Can Induce During Sex

1. Clitoral erections.

During oral sex, penetrative intercourse, or by utilizing a grinding action, you can give your girlfriend a clitoral orgasm with your fingers.

'The Welcome Method' is a terrific method to utilize if you want to give your wife a clitoral orgasm with your fingers.

2. Using the Deep Spot Method, Vaginal Orgasms

The greatest strategy to induce a vaginal orgasm in your girlfriend is to use the Deep Spot Method, a particular fingering technique. Women can experience many vaginal orgasms during a single sexual encounter since they are such intense physical sensations for them.

3. Vaginal Orgasms. Through Sexual Contact

These orgasms, which take place during penetrative intercourse, are extremely gratifying for a woman. She would undoubtedly think the sex was amazing if a man frequently causes her to have vaginal orgasms during the encounter.

4. An amalgam orgasm
A combined orgasm is one that happens as a result of two different forms of stimulation.

Licking your partner's clitoris and simultaneously massaging her G-Spot with your middle and index fingers is one of the greatest ways to achieve this.
makes them insane.
5. the strongest orgasm ever experienced by a woman.
Massage a woman's G-Spot with your finger in her anus to induce her first anal erection.

6 Nipple Orgasm

Some women can experience orgasm by just stimulating their nipples.

Some approaches for nipple orgasm might help a woman reach climax more regularly. The areola, which is very pigmented and surrounds the nipple, is rich with nerve endings that make the area a real vulnerable spot for women.

"The art of defeating a tiger with the strength of a fly" is the key to stimulating the nipples. When you translate this Chinese proverb to refer to female breasts, the emphasis is on the pleasure experienced.

Create a few circles around the nipple's peak before reaching it.

The recommended approach combines fluid motions with a gradual rise in pressure. Circular motions can be paired with gentle, and occasionally somewhat violent, pinches. A great first step to an orgasm is to lubricate the area with saliva to adjust the temperature.

If you combine your tongue with your hands' work, the pleasure is enhanced. She will build up energy prior to the ultimate explosion if you suck, softly bite, and contact the nipples with your tongue at various rates.

She will adore it if you softly tug her nipples with your lips.

Important: All sex gurus agree that the greatest advice is to communicate with your spouse in order to fully understand what she enjoys. In this manner, you will have crucial information straight from the source to make her scream the next time.

In fact, if you get good at this method and keep asking her what she likes and dislikes, she'll keep asking for more.

7. Orgasm with no physical contact

The strength of a man's speech and no physical contact of any kind induce is enhanced orgasm, which is frequently referred to as a "Mindgasm" by those who are familiar with it.

Mindgasms are incredibly strong and call for excellent, persistent DIRTY TALK.

As you can see, there are several methods for providing a lady with intense sexual pleasure. The majority of males decide to merely concentrate on the clitoris, guaranteeing that they never provide their wives with actually amazing sex.

How to get a man to orgasm

A male has the exact same requirements in the bedroom that a woman does. It's crucial to offer your boyfriend the same pleasure while you're in a relationship since failing to do so might lead to issues. Relationships need both men and women to put forth equal effort to maintain their half of the bargain when it comes to sexual activity.

You need a little assistance if you can't give your boyfriend a lot of pleasure. It's acceptable for you to feel bashful or ashamed when giving a man pleasure, but that's all about to change.

To assist you on your journey, you must master certain male orgasm strategies. You must discover what a man enjoys and detests in the bedroom. You will expand your repertoire of sexual acts so that you can always satisfy a man to the maximum.

Male orgasms are distinct from female orgasms in that males require far less stimulus and time to attain their peak sexual activity. This makes it simpler for women to win over guys, but it doesn't mean you should skimp on giving him everything you have to give. Attempting foreplay on your boyfriend is still a smart idea since it sets the stage for sex. It not only puts him in a good mood but also helps to put you in a good mood, which is significant. Equally, if not more so than the man's, is the importance of the woman's sexual mindset and being. The more invested you are, the more you

Men like forceful treatment, but if you take your time, you may teach him to view sex differently and alter the way he experiences an orgasm. Increasing the pressure inside his body is a terrific male orgasm strategy. Stop stimulating him just as he is ready to climax and don't let him release. As soon as you start stimulating him again, his pressure increases, and when he finally climaxes, it will be explosive and incredibly unforgettable for both of you.

Don't be scared to utilize your sexuality to dominate your partner in bed and to offer him a lot of pleasure. You'll feel content after doing this.

There are consequences beyond only your sex life when you lack sexual confidence in the bedroom. You aren't asserting your femininity or your potential for sexual power. Find out what you can do to change your intimate connection with your partner and yourself entirely starting now.

The benefits of a satisfying sex

Any love relationship must include sexual activity since it has both psychological and physiological advantages. It is a way to express intimacy, connect with your spouse, and keep your body and mind in good shape. Couples can show their love and desire for one another via physical contact. However, depending on the people involved and their unique wants and goals, the significance of sex in a relationship might change.

The physical and emotional connection that sex fosters in a relationship is among its most significant advantages. Sexual intercourse with your spouse may increase your sense of closeness and connection to them as well as promote sentiments of trust.

Regular sex has been found to alleviate stress, strengthen the immune system, and even cut your chance of developing certain diseases including prostate cancer and heart disease. Sex also produces endorphins, which may lift your spirits and make you happier all around.

1. It fosters intimacy and connection.

A stronger connection with your spouse may be made via sexual intimacy. In a way that no other activity can, it enables you to share who you are. Oxytocin, a hormone that encourages bonding and emotions of trust and closeness, is released during sexual activity. When you engage in sexual activity with your spouse, you forge a unique connection that may bolster your bond and make you feel closer to one another.

2. Enhances Physical Well-being.

Your physical health also depends on your sexual life. Maintaining a healthy weight,

lowering your risk of heart disease and stroke, and boosting your immune system may all be achieved with regular sexual activity. Endorphins, the body's natural painkillers, are also released.
They can aid in easing pain and encouraging relaxation. Additionally, it has been demonstrated that sexual engagement enhances sleep and lowers blood pressure, all of which are beneficial for general health.

3. Promotes Emotional Well-being

Additionally beneficial to your mental well-being, sex. Dopamine and serotonin, two feel-good chemicals that are released as a result, can help lessen stress, anxiety, and sadness. Additionally, engaging in sexual action fosters emotions of joy and pleasure, which can lift your spirits and increase your sense of closeness to your partner.

4. Enhances Self-Esteem: Engaging in sexual activity can boost self-esteem. It makes you feel wanted and beautiful, which can assist to increase your self-worth and confidence. You might feel more at ease in your own skin by having sex with a person who values and appreciates you.

5. Boosts Contentment in Relationships Finally, having sex is essential to a happy and healthy relationship. Regular sexual activity can improve a couple's sense of intimacy, connection, and relationship satisfaction. Building trust and understanding between spouses is made possible by the ability of partners to express their needs and wishes. Setting sex as a priority can help you and your spouse become closer and improve your overall relationship happiness. Sex is an essential component of a successful relationship

Conclusion

In conclusion, sexual intimacy is a crucial component of any love partnership. It improves both the body and the mind, fosters closeness and connections, and enhances general health and wellbeing. You will build a solid, wholesome, and lasting relationship by emphasizing sexual activity and being open to your spouse. Every relationship sex dynamics are crucial, but they are not the only thing that affect how well they work. A harmonious combination of emotional closeness, trust, respect, and sexual intimacy is necessary for a successful partnership.